Crystals and Gemstones

Guide to Healing Illnesses with the Power of Stones

various sources. Please consult a licensed professional before attempting any techniques outlined in this book.

By reading this document, the reader agrees that under no circumstances is the author responsible for any losses, direct or indirect, which are incurred as a result of the use of information contained within this document, including, but not limited to, —errors, omissions, or inaccuracies.

Table of Contents

Introduction: Understanding Crystals, their Healing Powers, and a Brief History

Crystals are formed under the surface of the earth over millennia. Crystals and gemstones are special rocks because the molecular structure within these rocks has repetitive patterns. The repetitive molecular patterns are formed depending on the heat, pressure, vibrational and other forms of energy these substances were subjected to over millions of years.

Therefore, it is right to assume that crystals have millennia-old universal energy trapped within them that can effectively be harnessed for healing and other purposes today. Crystals and gemstones have fascinated humankind from the beginning of time, and this intense fascination could be a result of one or more of the following reasons:

- Crystals are beautiful to look at. They dazzle in the sunlight, and the myriad colors of nature that they emanate can grab and hold anyone's attention.

- From ancient times, human beings have believed and leveraged the healing powers of these crystals.
- Crystals are flexible and dynamic and can be easily included into your spiritual enhancement regimen.

Healing with crystals and gemstones is not a new phenomenon. They have always been used by humankind since time immemorial. Amulets and talismans have always found a place in the history of human beings. Let us take a brief historical journey into the use of crystals for their healing and spiritually uplifting powers.

A Brief History of Crystals and Gemstones

Excavations in Singur, Russia have unearthed mammoth ivory beads that are believed to be more than 60,000 years old. Amulets made of Baltic amber that are considered to be over 30,000 years old, and amber beads over 10,000 years old have been excavated in certain parts of Britain.

Excavations of the graves of the Paleolithic Age (in present-day Belgium and Switzerland) threw up necklaces, bracelets and beads made from crystals. The Sinai Peninsular in Egypt has been the home of malachite mines for 4000 years ago.

The first recorded history of the use of crystals is from the Ancient Sumerian Civilization who used crystals and gemstones to create magic formulas and potions. The Ancient Egyptians were not far behind, and they wore clear quartz, emerald, turquoise and lapis lazuli as jewelry for health and protection purposes.

The Ancient Greeks also attributed multiple properties to many crystals and, in fact, many of the crystal names have their roots in the ancient Greek language. The word, 'crystal' itself means 'ice' in the Greek language because the ancient Greeks believed that water solidified and froze at such depths and under such tremendous pressure that it became permanently crystallized and could not revert to its former liquid state. Amethyst means 'not drunk' and was used to prevent hangovers and drunkenness.

Interestingly, some crystals were believed to have similar medicinal and healing properties by different and disparate civilizations separated by thousands of miles. For example, Jade was believed to have kidney-healing properties by the Chinese, the Mayan, and the Aztec Civilizations. Turquoise is worn for health and vitality and jasper calmness and health the world over.

Then, in the Middle Ages, crystals were banned by the church for various reasons. During the Renaissance periods, the probing intellectuals started looking for scientific reasons for the behavior and properties of crystals. Now, of course, crystals are not used extensively in the mainstream medical industry, but they continue to be used by believers for mental and physical healing and health.

Why and How Do Crystals Work?

Marcel Vogel was one of the first scientists who did some pioneering experiments with crystals and their healing powers. While he observed the growth of crystals under a microscope, he noticed that they took the form or the shape of whatever he was thinking about.

Based on these interesting and strange observations, Marcel Vogel postulated that the bonds between the molecules in the crystals had the power to continually assemble and reassemble to align with the thoughts and the mind of the observer. Further, he studied and tested the metaphysical power latent in the quartz crystal and concluded that it can store thoughts just like magnetic tapes record and store sound.

Albert Einstein believed that all things in the universe are composed of vibrational energy. These vibrational energies behave like sound waves in such a way that your thoughts align with everything else in your life, and vice versa. Therefore, the vibrational energies in the crystal have the power to amplify your thoughts.

Thoughts create vibrations in the universe, and therefore setting the right intention with your thoughts is a powerful tool to achieve happiness and well-being. A clear intention, goal, or purpose helps us identify with and understand our deepest desires and dreams. Additionally, focusing on thoughts to create the right intention increases our self-awareness and facilitates living 'in the moment.'

Intentions behave like magnets attracting resources and other elements in the universe that help in making our dreams a reality. Here are some tips on how to set intentions before you start working with crystals:

Decide what is important to you - Your values and intentions are the driving force in your life. In the absence of intentions and values, your life is bound to move haphazardly, and you will not find fulfillment. Therefore, take some time off from your hectic routine, and think about the things that matter to you the most.

Ask yourself which areas of your life need improvement – What aspects of your life need improvement? Are relationships an issue? Do you want to improve your health, spirituality, community and social life, career, or anything else?

Create specific intentions and goals – Decide what you want to achieve, when, and how. Also, identify the reason behind your intentions. Why do you want to do what you want to do?

Now, give life to your intentions – Some of the rituals using crystals require you to write down your intentions as if they are happening right now in your life. Fill your intentions with powerful emotions and feelings, and fill your mind with thoughts of your goals and intentions.

Certain crystals amplify these intentions, and by the law of attraction, you will be able to draw the required resources and energies from the universe to make your intentions become a reality.

Here is another way crystals work for our benefit. Our thoughts fill our minds preventing us from connecting with the universal energies that surround us. Crystals help in silencing our thoughts so that we can reconnect with the universal energy and feel rejuvenated and refreshed. Another critical lesson taught by crystals is patience. It took eons for crystals to trap the power of the earth and universe within their molecular systems. In the same way, we need to be patient and persist in our efforts to harness the healing powers of crystals.

Therefore, as you begin your journey to the wonderful world of crystals and their healing powers, remember to persist and be patient with yourself and the world around you. With practice, your ability to harness the healing power of crystals will improve slowly but surely.

Chapter One: Choosing the Right Crystals for You

Experts in the crystal world believe that you don't choose the crystal. The crystal chooses you. Yet, there is plenty of information and experience that has been passed through generations of believers of the power of crystal that it does make sense to learn as much as you can before taking your first step into this magical and mesmerizing world.

If you are choosing a crystal from a bricks-and-mortar store, all you need to do initially is to walk around the shop and look at all the crystals on display. It is highly likely that one or two stand out in your eyes, and you might really not be able to pinpoint a tangible reason for this phenomenon at that point in time. And yet, there will be a 'calling,' for want of a better word, where these 1-2 crystals appear almost as if they are trying to reach out to you. This is what crystal experts believe happens with all crystal choices.

Here are some general guidelines that could, perhaps, give you some insight into the 'process' that goes into making the right crystal choice.

Seek Help from the Universe

Yes, when you desire something deeply enough, the entire universe aligns with your desire and gives you multiple signs to help you in your search. Here are some tips to recognize signs sent by the universe:

Request for signs – Human beings are creatures of a powerful free will and the ability to think and visualize our needs. The spiritual capability inherent in each of us can recognize and receive guidance from the universe. You can ask for signs by making a little note of your request in your journal requesting signs. It could be something as simple as a thought that sparks in your mind or a simple prayer that comes to your lips. These are all powerful signs.

Become familiar with various ways that the universe connects with you – The language of the universe is different from that which you speak with your friends and family. The universal energy uses different ways to connect with you. It could be in the form of animals or numbers or colors or words from a wise elder in your home or even dreams that keep coming up in your life trying to tell you something. These are signs from the universe. Be sensitive to them, and familiarize yourself with them.

Acknowledge, accept, and act on these signs – When you acknowledge a sign that has been sent to you, the universe understands that you are now open and alert to receiving more such messages. Therefore, instead of ignoring these signs, acknowledge, accept and act on them with your body, mind and soul. The more you recognize and acknowledge signs transmitted to you, the more the universe can connect with you.

Seek Out Any Physical Reactions with Any Crystal

Take your non-dominant hand and pass it over different crystals. Sometimes, if the vibrational energy between your thoughts and the energy of the crystals resonate, then you could feel a 'tug' on your hand or palm. They are subtle but unmistakably physical reactions. Check out for such physical reactions to choose your crystal(s).

Identify the Crystal or Gemstone for Your Particular Problem

As a beginner, this could, perhaps, be your first option. What is the problem that you are trying to solve? Pick up a crystal, which is empowered with the property to solve this particular problem.

A good place to begin this learning is by understanding which part of your body needs healing. Each part of the body is identified with chakras or wheels of energy, and the vibrational energy of each chakra is aligned with the energy of certain crystals. Therefore, you can choose the crystal based on the chakra that needs healing.

Chakras and Their Significance to Our Well-Being

At this juncture, it makes sense to spend some time on the various chakras in the body, their energy purpose, and their corresponding crystals. Chakras with blocked energies or other functional problems can result in illnesses of the body and mind. Therefore, understanding each chakra, its position, and significance is important for healing. There are seven primary chakras in our body including:

The root chakra – Located at the base of your backbone in the region of the tailbone, the root chakra represents your grounding and foundational strength. The root chakra is responsible for survival issues such as finances, food, money, etc. It is associated with the color red.

A low level of energy in this chakra results in fearfulness and lack of self-confidence. Emotional and physical stability could also be hampered. An excessive amount of energy in the root chakra could result in an excessive feeling of attachment in a negative way such as clinging on to old and valueless belief systems that are hampering your physical, mental and intellectual growth.

Typically, red-colored crystals such as red jasper, hematite, smoky quartz, etc. help in healing and balancing the root chakra.

The sacral chakra – This chakra is situated in the lower abdomen about 2 inches below your navel and 2 inches inside. It is connected to your sexual and relationship energy. A healthy and balanced sacral chakra helps you maintain strong connections with others and facilitates new experiences with new situations and people. The sacral chakra is associated with wellbeing, plenitude, sexuality, and pleasure.

When the energy levels in the sacral chakra are lower than needed, then you could feel emotionally stifled and sexually inactive. You could disconnect with people around you. On the other hand, an overactive sacral chakra could lead to mood disorders such as bipolarity, depression, anxiety, etc.

The sacral chakra is connected to the color, and the crystals that can help in its healing are coral and orange calcite, orange carnelian, citrine, and orange aventurine.

The solar plexus chakra – Located in the upper abdomen, this chakra's energy represents your self-confidence. It reflects your ability to control your life. The emotional issues controlled by the solar plexus chakra include self-esteem and self-confidence.

A lower-than-needed energy level in this chakra could result in a feeling of low self-esteem, a feeling of being invisible, and not allowing your personal power to be active. An overactive solar plexus chakra could result in a domineering, compulsive, and obsessive personality.

Yellow is the color of the solar plexus chakra. The crystals that help to heal and balance this chakra are pyrite stones (that hold the power of the golden sun), golden Lemurian, agate stone, and tiger's eye.

The heart chakra – The energy of the heart chakra reflects your ability to give and receive love. It is located just above the heart in the center of the chest. It deals with inner peace, love, and joy. The heart chakra helps you to feel; an important element needed for all kinds of healing. A healthy and balanced heart chakra radiates love for yourself and for others around you.

A blocked or imbalanced heart chakra will make feel detached from the world around you, from people who love and care for you, and even from self-love. This chakra is associated with the color green. Crystals of the heart chakra include aventurine, amazonite, jade, malachite, and rose quartz.

The throat chakra – Located at the throat, this chakra reflects our communication ability. It deals with expressions of feelings and articulation. It also represents the expression of truth.

An imbalanced throat chakra results in compromised communication capabilities. You will find yourself unable to express your emotions and feelings. You will feel trapped. The color of the throat chakra is blue.

Crystals that promise to heal the throat chakra include sodalite, Angelite, lapis lazuli, aquamarine, azurite, and turquoise.

The third eye chakra – Located between the eyes on the forehead, the third eye chakra reflects our ability for focus and concentrate and helps us to see the bigger picture. It is associated with imagination, intuition, wisdom, extrasensory perceptions, and our ability to think through various things and take appropriate decisions.

A balanced and healthy third eye chakra helps you depend on your inner senses and intuition for guidance in various decision-making aspects of your life. The third eye chakra helps you include the powers of your soul along with your intellect and emotions to make beneficial decisions. A blocked third eye chakra could make you feel fearful and uncertain about the future of your life.

The color of the third eye chakra is purple. Crystals that are useful for healing this chakra include fluorite, shungite, amethyst, lapis lazuli, and quartz.

The crown chakra – Located at the top of your head, the crown chakra is associated with your spiritual ability. It deals with balancing the outer and inner beauty of the body and mind, and your relationship with spirituality, inner consciousness and bliss.

A balanced and healthy crown chakra represents your desire to enhance yourselves spiritually. It reflects in your ability to empathize and a deep connection with the Supreme Being. An unbalanced or blocked crown chakra could result in your inability to reach out for higher wisdom resulting in constant worry and anxiety despite being materially well-off.

The color of the crown chakra is white or purple. Crystals that heal this chakra are clear quartz, amethyst, charoite, howlite, and selenite.

Therefore, when you walk into a crystal store or shop online for them, you can choose your crystal based on which chakra you want to be healed. Picking the right crystal is a combination of your intuitive powers and knowledge that you gain.

Chapter Two: Important and Popular Crystals and Their Healing Properties

The world of crystals and gemstones is so large that it can overwhelm a beginner. There are a mind-boggling number of crystals available on the market so that deciding what you want can be quite intimidating. This chapter is dedicated to giving you some basic insights into some of the crystals that are both popular and important for healing.

The first 7-10 crystals are must-haves. The others that follow can be looked at once you delve deeper into this amazing and magical world and discover for yourself what you really want. Let's dive right in.

Clear Quartz – The Master Healer

This crystal is a great first choice for a beginner. It is the most iconic representative of the quartz family of crystals and is abundantly available everywhere on Earth because it can develop in any kind of environmental circumstance. Having been on this planet for so many eons, clear quartz has found its way into nearly tribe and community's folklore.

Quartz has its etymological roots in the Greek word for 'ice.' The ancient Greek philosophers and wise men like Theophrastus and others believed that this beautiful transparent stone was some form of permanent ice. They believed that water had solidified so deeply that it could not revert back to its liquid state, and this kind of 'permanently solidified water' was called quartz.

Clear quartz is called the master healer because of its amazing versatility and its ability to smoothen out energy flows in all the chakras. It can be programmed for any purpose. Clear quartz cannot only direct its own energy for effective healing but can also enhance the healing power of other crystals. It brings clarity to your thoughts and enhances the strength and brightness of your aura.

Different cultures had different reasons for using clear quartz for healing. The Japanese believed that clear quartz was the 'perfect jewel' because it represented space, patience and purity. Tribal cultures in North American offered clear quartz as food along with other offerings to their gods.

Some of the South American and Australian cultures have woven their origin or creational stories around clear quartz. They believed that creator life is a cosmic serpent that was coiled and held in clear quartz. In some other South American and Central American cultures, clear quartz was sacred because they believed that, like an urn, it held the spirits of their ancestors. These people believed that the metaphysical properties of clear quartz could heal the illnesses of their cattle.

Clear quartz is an essential crystal needed during crystal-based healing for its programmability and amplification properties. Although this crystal is not connected to any one particular Zodiac sign, it is believed to have the power to temper down the power desires of the Leos and the adamant nature of the Capricorns.

Tiger's Eye – The Stone for Confidence

The tiger's eye is a perfect start to build self-esteem and confidence. This beautiful golden brown tiger-stripped stone is replete with a masculine kind of energy. It is the ultimate power crystal and can help you free yourself from self-doubt created either by your own past failures or by jealous people in your life. It is also excellent for grounding purposes.

This gemstone is also referred to as chatoyancy, which is French for cat, and if including in your daily meditation can fuel your deepest passions. The tiger's eye resonates with the solar plexus chakra and is connected with making money. It teaches you the most essential aspect of economics, which is 'with increased productivity comes increased wealth and money.'

The tiger's eye stone empowers you with the motivation needed to make things happen and realize your dreams and desires. Moreover, this crystal helps you balance your power by living a life of honesty and integrity to achieve success. After all, the tiger is the largest cat in the world, and yet it allows the lion to be the king of the jungle.

The tiger's eye can be your personal life coach who gives you the strength and motivation to come out of your dream world and work hard to make those dreams come true. It empowers you with risk-taking capabilities and drives you to move out of your comfort zone; both key elements for success, expansion, and growth.

Amethyst – The Psychic Powerhouse

Although suitable for most novices in the crystal world, it is important to keep in mind that this beautiful violet crystal with a name as lilting as amethyst has great powers to develop and expand your psychic capabilities.

It is found abundantly in Bolivia, Brazil, Africa, Mexico, Canada, and other parts of Europe and the US. Despite its wide prevalence, amethyst is one of the most revered crystals since time immemorial. The ancient Romans and Greeks associated amethyst with luxury and, therefore, the highly regarded stone was found in royal rings, crowns and scepters.

Catholic clergymen wore amethyst because they believed it had the powers to inspire celibacy and piety. The ancient Greeks believed that the power to inhibit intoxication was bestowed on this crystal by Bacchus, the Greek God of wine, fertility, and agriculture, and therefore, this stone was worn to prevent hangovers and drunkenness. The Chinese Feng Shui philosophers associated amethyst with wealth, and if placed in the wealth corner of the house, can bring in prosperity.

Amethyst is connected with the crown chakra and is believed to help you connect with your deepest spiritual powers, and if you are not prepared to handle this situation, then it could unnerve you a bit. And yet, amethyst is the perfect beginner's choice for protection and to cleanse your body and surroundings of all kinds of negative energies.

Amethyst can help clear negative energies resulting from anxiety and stress. It helps in purification of the mind and building your spiritual and psychic powers. Many people meditate with an amethyst held in their palms to rid themselves of confusion and darkness.

Amethyst is an effective healer for work-related anxieties and stress and for stress associated with the lack of money, wealth and abundance. Your communication and intuitive powers can also be enhanced with the healing power of the amethyst crystal. Keeping an amethyst in your office space will help you include your intuitive powers with intellect and knowledge to take tough but effective decisions for improved business success. An amethyst placed in the family room will increase familial bonding and frees up the atmosphere for open and honest conversations among loved ones.

Hematite – The Bouncer Crystal

This powerful deflector of negative energies protects you from psychic attacks. It deflects negative energy aimed at you and transfers it to Mother Earth for healing. Therefore, it is called as the Bouncer Crystal. If for any inexplicable reason you feel drawn to hematite, then it is quite likely that you are in search of grounding and stability.

The minute you touch a hematite crystal, you will feel centered and calm. It is the perfect crystal to cleanse and clear the root chakra, and subsequently, achieve the calming effects of grounding yourself. Hematite offers an immense sense of stability.

The hematite crystal absorbs all the toxic emotions and energies that are holding you back from achieving your potential. It clears all negative energies connected to stress, worry and anxiety. By grounding you to Mother Earth and increasing the power of your root chakra, hematite enhances self-confidence and power during stressful times.

In addition to healing your mental worries and stresses, hematite is known to cleanse and clear your circulatory system. Found in abundance in Australia, hematite got its name because of the red color rendered by the high content of iron in this stone. "Haima' is the Latin word for blood, and that explains the etymology of hematite. Hematite is perfect to calm your troubled mind by simply grounding you and strengthening your root chakra.

Rose Quartz – The Mother of all Crystals

Gentle, soothing and calming properties characterize the rose quartz crystal. It is a great healer of emotional pain. It opens and clears the energy blockages in the heart chakra enhancing your capability of loving everyone including yourself. Connected to the heart chakra, this is the perfect self-love stone for beginners.

A gemstone for the hopeless romantic from time immemorial rose quartz has been a permanent fixture in love rituals for centuries. Like the clear quartz, this is also a member of the quartz family and is primarily made of silicon dioxide. The soft, pink color is a result of irradiation as well as the minute inclusions of pink-colored fibers within the stone.

The irradiation effect is why it is essential to keep rose quartz out in the sun to prevent it from losing its natural pink color. The rose quartz is found in plenty all over the world, and largely in Madagascar, Brazil, South Africa, and India. The early Egyptian, Roman and Greek civilizations used rose quartz talismans to represent a negotiated deal.

The symbol of love was first attached to this beautiful pink stone by Roman and Greek myths. It is believed that the blood of Aphrodite and her lover Adonis is what gives this crystal a pink color. Another legend says that Eros, the Greek God of love gave the rose quartz to human beings as a symbol of love.

While the romantic kind of love is what is popularly connected with the rose quartz crystal, in reality, this crystal represents unconditional love. The rose quartz can take your consciousness to a higher level thereby empowering you to accept and give love unconditionally. It helps you look at conflicts and fights in different perspectives, which, in turn, helps you, forgive and move on in the relationship.

Additionally, rose quartz awakens the spirit of self-love and self-compassion and empowers you to forgive yourself too. This magical gemstone cleans toxins in the form of negative emotions and energies from your body and mind. Hold rose quartz close to your heart to begin the unbridled and unconditional journey of love.

Turquoise – Another Master Healer

Believed to be the spiritual energy bridge between human beings and the divine, turquoise is another master healer among crystals. Since ancient times, turquoise has been worn for its ability to bring good luck to and protect the wearer. It was worn by the likes of King Tutankhamen and Queen Cleopatra for its amazing protective ability.

Moreover, if you give or receive this beautiful blue-green crystal as a gift, then its healing powers increase multifold. Turquoise is also effective to improve communication as it helps you speak the truth always, irrespective of the repercussions. Turquoise symbolizes the oceans of the world.

The warriors in the ancient times wore an amulet embedded with turquoise before starting off on any battle for the crystal's personal protection capabilities. The Aztecs too wore this crystal on battle gear and ceremonial masks. Persian legends hold that when turquoise reflects the moonlight, then it is supposed to bring good luck.

Today, turquoise is used to heal wounded hearts and to smooth out chronic forms of stress. This crystal promotes energetic flow empowered by the highest energy frequency namely love. Additionally, like quartz, turquoise is highly versatile and can be programmed for specific healing intentions.

You can program your turquoise crystal as a good luck charm, to realign and balance your chakras, or clear the spiritual path to reach higher levels of consciousness. Hold it in your hand as you perform your daily meditation, and feel uplifted by its calming and soothing effect brought on by the world's most beloved emotional food; love.

Citrine – The Prosperity Crystal and the Light Maker

This orange-hued crystal is known for its ability to attract wealth and prosperity into your life. Closely connected to the solar plexus chakra, it is also known to boost self-confidence and self-worth. Citrine can clear any aura of negativities resulting in an increased intensity of positivity.

Citrine oozes light energy and emanates joy and positivity. Citrine gets its name from the French word for lemon and is undoubtedly connected to the sun and the joy it is capable of spreading. It is found abundantly and in its natural state in Spain, Brazil, Russia, Africa, Madagascar, the US, and other countries too.

Citrine has been used to increase the aura and beauty of ornaments since ancient times. It found its way into Scottish men's wear in the form of shoulder poaches, kilt pins, and to brighten swords and daggers, thanks to Queen

Victoria's affinity for this yellow-hued beautiful crystal.

Citrine's healing powers lie in its capabilities to clear energy blockages in the sacral, solar plexus, and the third chakras to boost your creativity and spiritual progress. It increases your sexual and fertility energies as well. Citrine placed in the bedroom can increase intimacy, and when placed in the office space can bring in prosperity and success. In children's rooms, citrine brings in a sense of security through the golden light of the sun.

Citrine being the crystal of happiness and sunlight holds no negativity and is almost purely positive. It reminds you to live in the present moment instead of worrying about your past or future.

Bloodstone – The Energy Crystal

Bloodstone represents vitality, courage, strength, and purification.

Known for its ability to overcome lethargy, this energy-inducing crystal purifies blood too. It helps to overcome negative thoughts and feelings and is a great energy booster.

Additionally, the uplifting and purifying bloodstone crystal increases drive and motivation and boosts enthusiasm too.

During the Middle Ages, the red spots in the red-green stone were believed to be the blood of Christ, which seemed to render the crystal with magical powers. The green color of the crystal was thought to represent the power of the Earth, and the wearer of bloodstone is protected from negative effects and negative energy.

Summarily, bloodstone works to stabilize and ground your physical and mental powers while increasing your courage, strength, and determination to take on and overcome challenges that obstruct your pathway to success.

Carnelian – The Creativity and Action Crystal

Carnelian has the power to remove energy blocks in your mind that are preventing your creativity reaching its potential. Such negative energies dominate your mind and you feel burned out and completely uninspired. The powerful orange hue of the carnelian crystal sparks your passion and drives you to move ahead. It is an action that motivates and compels you to find joy and happiness by pushing you to realize your dreams and desires.

In the ancient times, carnelian was found on breastplate armor because of its ability to render courage and strength to the warrior who carried it. Whenever you feel stifled by stage fright, hold a carnelian in your hand, and watch the fear dissolve into nothingness.

The early Egyptians always wore carnelian on their bodies because they believed in its power to restore and renew strength and vitality. Today, carnelian stone is prescribed for increasing personal power, creativity and courage. Carnelian also diminishes the power of negative emotions such as jealousy, fear, anger, and resentment so that you are more in control of your life. With the power of carnelian on your side, you feel calm, healthy, strong, and happy.

Celestite – The Stress-Relieving Crystal

The Latin word for celestial (or heavenly) is 'caelestis' which is the root of the name of the celestite crystal. The divine blue color of celestite inspires calmness and tranquility. You simply need to gaze at this beautiful hue to feel balanced and peaceful.

When you place this crystal on any part of your body, the tension in that area will be released, and your muscles will feel relaxed. When placed in your bedroom, celestite can help you get a restful sleep. The celestite crystal is perfect for the chaotic mind. The feelings associated with this crystal are serenity, calmness, uplifting, and soothing.

If you are an impulsive person, then celestite is the perfect crystal to cool you down. Taking rash decisions or behaving rashly in the heat of the moment can only worsen the situation. If you feel your temper is getting in the way of the clarity of your thoughts, then celestite is the crystal to reach out to.

Selenite – The Liquid Light

This gorgeous looking crystal is sometimes referred to as Satin Spar for the milky sheen that radiates from its surface. Selenite is used extensively by metaphysical healers to improve well-being and for protection. It is found abundantly across the globe including the USA, Mexico, Australia, and Greece. However, most healers prefer the Mexican selenite for effective healing work.

Selenite is a very soft stone, and therefore, quite flexible. It gets its name from the Greek Moon Goddess, Selene, for this reason; when the crystal reflects moonlight, it looks like a drop of the moon has landed on the Earth. Although selenite is very soft, its metaphysical healing powers are phenomenal. Its most useful property is the rock's ability to help you activate your higher levels of consciousness by aligning all your chakras.

Selenite has the power to compel honesty and integrity in people who are under its aura. It clears energy blockages and allows the vibrations to flow through your body and mind as smoothly as a liquid. Healers use selenite to connect with guardian angels and spirit guides. These crystals can also multiply the effects of other crystals when they are used in tandem. Using selenite in the crystal grid (more about crystal grids in Chapter Four) in your home can help to keep out toxic influences.

Tourmaline – The Energy Cleanser

Tourmaline is an excellent cleanser of energy fields. It facilitates the removal of negative thought patterns and other forms of negative energies. It acts like a bodyguard saving you from the world's negativities. Known for its powerful capability to absorb electromagnetic radiation, tourmaline is perfect to keep near computers and other electronic devices to keep your body and mind safe from the harmful effects of radiations.

Simply place a tumbled stone of tourmaline in a bowl of water in your main living area, and you will feel a noticeable reduction in negativities and prickly thought patterns that were hitherto thwarting your progress. Its natural black color allows this energy-absorbing crystal to consume all wavelengths of all colors. Tourmaline is great to use when you are overcome by phobias and fears as it will simply ingest your anxieties like a sponge.

When you wear tourmaline on your body like in a piece of jewelry or accessory, it is like wearing a sign that tells the negative powers of the universe that they cannot cross the line.

Carrying it in your pocket will ensure you don't pick up other people's negative aura. Connected with the root chakra, tourmaline helps you feel secure and grounded.

Onyx – The Crystal for Letting Go

The onyx is known for its amazing ability to root out fear from your system. Fear is one of the most toxic and debilitating emotions, and when you let go of fear, there is nothing to stop you from reaching your fullest potential. When you let go of fears, you find the courage to fall into the deepest depths of your soul helping you find things that otherwise remain completely hidden.

The onyx crystal has three bands of colors including white, gray, and black. White is the color of the day sky, black is the color of the night sky, and gray is the color of the dusk and pre-dawn skies. The powers of healing and magic are most intense during the dusk and pre-dawn times when change is taking place at the optimal intensity. These three colors of the onyx crystal represent the interconnectedness of the black-and-white of the world.

Onyx is highly effective to heal anxieties and worries as it soothes and calms the frazzled and frenetic thoughts of your mind. You can use it to heal cracks that keep appearing in your work-life balance. And when you feel fear, reach out for that onyx in your crystal box. Hold it to your heart, and send a wish to the universe to be relieved of this debilitating fear. And watch your fears dissolve into nothingness.

Calcite – The Energy Amplifier

Two of the most commonly used calcite stones are green and orange, although this gemstone is available in a huge variety of colors and types. The combination of these two calcite crystals has the power to magnify and amplify the energy of the other crystals used in the healing process. Calcite comes from the Greek word for 'lime.'

Green calcite, by itself, is excellent for attracting prosperity and good fortune. In addition, the color green helps you connect with the natural world. When you meditate with a green calcite in your hand, you will discover ways to draw energy from Earth's life source. Moreover, the soothing green color will keep reminding you of the immense power latent in nature and will teach you to be grateful for this beautiful life in the midst of magical nature.

Jade – The Lucky Charm Crystal

Jade is deeply connected with the heart chakra. It is the ultimate good luck charm, and its powerful vibrational energy brings in abundance and prosperity into your life. Jade was one of the most sought-after gemstones in the Chinese civilization, and this tradition continues even to this day. Jade stones were used on the crowns and tombstones of Chinese emperors.

The green color of the jade crystal reflects the pristine and beautiful vegetation of Mother Earth. In the same way as green plants can provide food for the entire world by harnessing the power of sunlight, the jade crystal can harness the metaphysical powers of the sunlight for your well-being, growth, and vitality.

Jade is also the crystal of eternal youth and is used extensively in facial and skin treatments.

People use jade rollers over their faces to allow the natural rejuvenating power of jade to smoothen out wrinkles and restore the youthfulness of their facial skin.

Meditate with a jade crystal in your hand, and leverage the power of good fortune as it enters your life. Jade crystal also helps you feel gratitude for all the good things in your life.

Amazonite – The Optimism Crystal

Reflecting the verdant foliage of the beautiful, lush Amazonian region, amazonite is also a great stone to draw good luck to your life. Amazonite is referred to as the anti-anxiety medication in the world of crystals. Amazonite is called as the 'hope stone,' as it helps to fill your heart and mind with a can-do attitude.

It has the power to clear away and cleanse all the negative psychic debris accumulated in your system. Hold it close to your heart, and watch all the toxic emotions leaving your body and mind leaving you stress-free and filled with optimism for the future.

The crystals mentioned in this chapter offer you only a glimpse into the wonderful and powerful world of crystals and gemstones. First, experiment with these crystals, and as your intuitive power and knowledge of the world of universal vibrational energy progresses, you can delve deeper.

Chapter Three: Taking Care of Crystals

Once you received a crystal, you become its guardian. It is your duty to purify its energies and keep it from getting corrupted and unusable. The reason for having to take care of crystals is because they have the power to absorb all kinds of energies around them including the negative ones. Therefore, cleansing, charging, programming, and other aspects need to be done so that your crystals are clean, clear and add value to your life.

There are primarily two parts to taking care of crystals and they are:

- Cleansing
- Recharging
- Programming

Cleansing Your Crystals

As mentioned earlier, crystals absorb energies from their surroundings. Cleansing them will facilitate the removal of negative energies so that they are ready to be charged and programmed for any specific purpose. The first time you need to cleanse your crystal is as soon as you get it for the first time, irrespective of whether it was gifted to you or you purchased it yourself.

After that, you must cleanse your crystal regularly depending on how often you use it and for what purpose. The crystals you wear or have around in your house need to be cleansed more regularly than those you use only occasionally for healing purpose. The crystals used on a daily basis are interacting with other surrounding energies at varying frequencies. Moreover, you will also know when your crystal needs cleansing. For example:

- Most crystals will lose their luster if you have not cleansed them.
- Quartz crystal will become cloudy instead of clear and bright which is its natural profile.
- Some crystals will be heavier and denser than before; it will seem that they are carrying an extra burden, which is nothing but the negative energies that they have absorbed.
- If you are wearing it on your body, then you will notice that it is not emitting the same vibrational energy that it was giving out before.

- If you have used your crystal(s) for a particularly intense energy situation such as an illness or a trauma, then cleansing of your crystal(s) after the session becomes important.
- You will also need to cleanse your crystal before reprogramming it for a different purpose.

Methods of Cleansing – There are different ways of cleansing your crystals. Some of them are described below. Try all of them, and identify which one works best for a particular gemstone as each crystal calls for a different cleansing method for optimum efficiency. Also, cleansing methods are person-specific, and therefore, try many methods, and choose what works for you and your crystal(s) the best.

Before you start off, it is important that you clear your own mind, and create a strong intention for the cleansing process. Crystals hold vibrational energies that are bound to get altered and affected by the impurities and other forms of discords they experience during their entire life cycle. Therefore, cleansing crystals calls for a strong intention to ensure they achieve a clear and pure state.

Here is a small ritual to get the right intention before the cleansing process. Hold the crystal(s) in your hand, and imagine them immersed in a white light. Visualize all the unwanted energies being spirited away into oblivion. Imagine your crystal(s) in a re-energized, natural, and pure state. Ask the universe to help restore your gemstones to their original and full energy potential.

Remain in this position for a little while or until you feel satisfied with your efforts at getting the right intention. And finally, pray and ask all the energies in the universe to facilitate the transformation of your crystal(s) into divine love and light.

After your mind is clear with the cleansing intention, clear the room using sage, bells, or even a simple mantra. This clearing refers to clearing negative energies. Of course, ensure the cleansing space is clear of physical clutter as well. The cleansing process is a ritual, and for any ritual to achieve success, you need to have a calm, peaceful, and serene atmosphere both mentally and physically.

Cleansing with flowing water – Water is a universal healer, and crystals and water have a long and old legacy. They work very well with each other, and therefore, using water to cleanse your crystal is one of the easiest and most effective methods. Here is what you can do:

- Hold the crystal under water. Although a river, ocean, rainwater, or natural spring is preferred, in a modern urban setting, this may not be possible. So, you can hold your gemstones under running tap water.
- Imagine the pure water removing all the negativities trapped inside the crystal. Imagine the energy and frequency disruptions within the crystal structure being smoothened out, and the negativities dissolving in the water and being eliminated.
- Use a little sea salt to rub over the crystal, and again place it under water for the salt to be cleansed away too.
- Let your gemstones dry out naturally under sunlight.

An important word of caution; some crystals cannot withstand being cleansed in water. For example, selenite will simply dissolve. Therefore, research your crystal and choose your method wisely. Also, remember to use cold running water. Do not use warm or hot water for cleansing purposes.

Cleansing with salt water – Some types (not all) are cleansed thoroughly with salt water. You can either choose to use sea water or plain water mixed with sea salt. If you cannot get sea salt, then normal cooking salt is fine too. Fill a glass bowl with water, dissolve some salt, and let your crystals lie fully submerged inside for 1-24 hours depending on the crystal, and the duration of the elapsed time since the last time you cleansed it.

After you remove the crystal from the salt water, ensure you thoroughly clean it in cool, refreshing running water to completely remove all traces of salt. The salt water used to cleanse the crystal should be discarded as it will have absorbed all the accumulated unwanted and negative energies from the crystals.

Cleansing with moonlight – The moon's energy frequencies are empowered for purification. The moonlight's cleansing capabilities have been harnessed by crystal healers from time immemorial. The moon radiates feminine energy, which can help in emotional and spiritual healing as well. Simply place your crystals under the moonlight either on a full moon or new moon day, and allow them to harness the moon's powerful energy frequencies.

Cleansing with sunlight – The power of the sun and its radiating light is as powerful as the moon. It would be naïve not to harness this amazing energy of the star of our solar system. Unlike the moon, the sun's energy frequencies are more masculine than feminine.

Place your crystals under the direct sunlight and allow the power of the radiant light to smoothen our energy wrinkles within the stones and eliminate all negativities from within.

Cleansing with snow – For those unfortunate enough to have access to blessed, beautiful snow, it can be an amazing crystal cleanser. Putting your crystals in snow is a fast and powerful method to cleanse and clear them of all negative and burdening energies.

Cleansing with earth – When you bury your crystals in the warmth of Mother Earth, you are effectively sending them back to their home. And nothing can soothe and cleanse more than a mother's love. All forms of lingering negativities will be cleared out of your favorite crystals. You can bury your crystals for 3, 7 or 11 days for the best cleansing effect. The power of your crystals will be completely reset and rejuvenated.

Cleansing with smoke – Smudging is a cleansing process where you use the smoke of sage, lavender, cedar, sweetgrass, copal, or other naturally-empowered sacred herbs to cleanse the surroundings. Smudging is also an effective cleansing method for crystals.

First, light the herbs and let them burn. After the flames die down, smoke will be created from the embers. Pass your crystals through this smoke while visualizing the negative energies being cleared away from them. Using smoke for cleansing is especially good for crystals embedded in jewelry. Such items could potentially corrode if you tried using water.

Cleansing with rock salt – Place your gemstones in a bed of salt for about 1-2 days.

This helps in the purification of the crystal's energy matrix.

Cleansing with sound – The power of certain sound frequencies has the power to cleanse and charge. The tinkle of a bell is one such sound energy. Just tinkle a bell close to your crystal(s), and visualize your gemstones being cleared of all negativities. Similarly, the sound of your voice and other sacred chants are used for charging and programming.

Cleansing with other crystals – A few crystals actually do not need any cleansing or clearing. Moreover, their energy frequencies are so unique that these crystals can help to clear and cleanse other crystals. Such rare treasures in the crystal world include carnelian, selenite, kyanite, amethyst, etc.

Place all your crystals under a slab of selenite, and you can rest assured that they will be cleared and cleansed of all negative energies. You can also use a cluster of amethyst in this way.

Recharging Your Crystals

Recharging of crystals typically happens when you cleanse them because the elements for cleansing also help to recharge your crystal's energy frequencies. However, you can cleanse and recharge separately too. After you finish cleansing your gemstones, create a new intention to recharge them with renewed energy.

Hold your crystals in your hand, and visualize a beam of a bright, white light entering them, and renewing the power of the crystal matrix. Hold this picture until you are satisfied with the strength of your intention, and begin your recharging process. Here is a quick summary to help you:

- Place your crystals under the bright and beautiful light of the sun. A sunbath renders an amazing glow to your crystals as their energy levels are restored to their full potential. Placing the crystals on the earth to receive sunlight will enhance the recharging process.
- Place your gemstones under the powerful moonlight on a full moon. Renewed energy will penetrate the crystals by the effect of the gentle moonlight.

- You can place your crystals in dynamic weather conditions such as a thunderstorm. This method will empower your gemstone with an amazing electromagnetic charge.
- An amethyst cluster is a great crystal charger, especially those that are etched in jewelry and small-sized crystals for which other charging methods mentioned above may not be suitable.

Your gemstones are work best and their energies remain ever fresh when they out in the open. Avoid using artificial materials to place your crystals in your office or your home. Use natural materials such as silk or velvet. Additionally, your crystals are fragile and can chip or break. Therefore, it is essential that you handle them with care. Carry your crystals in velvet, cotton, satin, or silk holders or bags.

Precautions to be Taken While Storing Your Crystals

Always store your gemstones in a clean and dry place. Exposure to moisture and dust can damage certain types of crystals. Also, if you live in a coastal area, then your crystals need to be protected against excessive exposure to salt air.

There could be some gemstones, which you would have bought with a lot of love, and you may have spent a lot of money too. For such pieces, it would be best if you stored them in boxes made of good-quality plastic or any other acid-free and inert materials to prevent any kind of chemical reactions between the crystal and the container.

For small pieces of crystals, buy yourself a good-sized box with multiple compartments, preferably lined with velvet or silk. Each crystal can be kept in one little compartment. This will look good and each gemstone will be nicely protected too. Keeping all together in one bunch can result in the harder and bigger crystals chipping and damaging the smaller and softer ones.

Also, avoid using cotton pads or balls as some kind of cushion because the fibers can stick to the corners of your special gemstones resulting in disrupting the energy frequencies. Tumbled stones or other polished items can be kept anywhere without much fuss.

Remember every specimen of crystal you have is unique. It is mined at specific geographic locations and has a unique geologic and genetic background. Once damaged and lost, you can never really replace the identical crystal with the exact same set of energy frequency. Crystals are divine treasures gifted to us by nature and Mother Earth, and therefore taking care of them is our duty and responsibility.

Programming Crystals

Programming a crystal is a ritual in which you assign special powers to your crystal to help you achieve a specific task or job. You could program your crystal to help you with your work, to help you in your relationships, to attract prosperity and abundance, to attract love, etc. You could program one crystal for each of these intentions and place them in strategic locations either at home or in your workplace.

Another useful program to input into a crystal is to help you to recall your dreams at night. Many times, the universe sends out powerful signs through dreams. And sadly, we don't make enough effort to try and recall our dreams except for the ones that really scare us. Program a crystal with this particular task, and keep it under your pillow. In the morning, hold the crystal in your palm as you try to recall your dreams as vividly as you can.

So, how do you program a gemstone? Here are a few helpful steps you can follow:

- First, decide what help you seek from the crystal.
- Choose a crystal that you are drawn to for this task, and ask if the gemstone is willing to partner with you in your endeavor. If the crystal's intentions are not aligned with yours, then you will get a definite sign of resistance for a 'No' answer. And, it is quite easy to discern the negative answer from a crystal. Positive answers, on the other hand, are tricky to determine. Many times, it is a neutral feeling you get when you put forward the willingness question to the crystal.
- Once you have chosen the right crystal, hold it first to your heart chakra, and then to your third eye chakra. Now, with a clear mind and intent, visualize your task or project being projected into the crystal. Extend this imagination outward until you see your heart, eye, and mind forming a triangle and locking your intent.
- Lastly, state your purpose aloud for the energies of the universe to hear.

- Give thanks to the crystal for its willingness to transmit your desire through its energy frequency

As you delve deeper into the realm of crystals, you will discover your own special powers of connecting with the energy frequency of crystals, and use the resultant resonating power for your own good and for that of others. Crystals are a boon to us, and we have to treat them with the utmost respect.

Chapter Four: Placement of Crystals for Everyday Benefits

In the world of crystals, everything and everyone is connected to each other and one another. Everything in the universe is nothing but a form of vibrational energy. The energies of different things and different people work at different frequencies, and when these frequencies resonate, then the result is optimum harmony, joy, and happiness.

Crystals have the power to work their magic and bring together the connecting frequencies to create harmony and health, and consequently, positive change. And that is the reason why crystals are powerful tools to heal, harmonize and eliminate negative energies within and outside of you. Here are some practical ways you can use crystals easily for effective healing and happiness.

1. ***Keep a crystal in your proximity right through the day***

Determine what kind of healing you want. What kind of frequency shift are you seeking in your vibrational energy? Based on these answers, choose the appropriate crystal. Cleanse it using one of the methods discussed in Chapter Three. Then, program the crystal for your specific purpose by creating the right intent using the following steps:

- Hold the crystal in your hand.
- Next, think of the problems for which you are seeking help from the crystals. Bring forth all the feelings and thoughts connected with your desired outcome.
- Imagine the outcome has already taken place, and you are enjoying its benefits.
- Transfer these positive thoughts into the crystal and imagine a white light passing through it and locking your purpose within the gemstone.
- Thank the crystal for helping you.
- The crystal's vibrational energy is now programmed to align with yours.

Now, keep this programmed crystal in your pocket or around your neck. Keep it on your body until you feel and believe that the gemstone's vibrational energy field has entered your own aura, and the combined energy fields are resonating effects are helping to bring about positive changes. Remember to cleanse and reprogram this crystal regularly to refresh, renew, and recharge its vibrational energy.

2. ***Keep a crystal under your pillow every night***

Crystals with vibrational energies suited for relaxation and restfulness are perfect to be placed under your pillow each night. For example, black tourmaline is a great gemstone that helps to remove all the harsh, frenetic and negative vibes and energies you might have absorbed during the day.

These negativities could be in any form ranging from the excessive exposure to harmful electromagnetic waves of electronic devices to the negative aura of people you would have interacted with throughout the day. Other gemstones are helpful in healing the physical and mental wounds received during the day include spirit quartz, selenite, Jasper, and amethyst.

Amethyst is also helpful if you have problems recalling your dreams. Remember the universe employs dreams to send you signs, and it would be unfortunate if you could not recall your dreams. Other crystals that can help in this include dream quartz (a greenish-pink colored gemstone that is difficult to find and expensive too) and hemimorphite (a beautiful blue stone that reminds you of a gorgeous icy glacier).

3. *Place crystals in strategic places in your home and office*

For example, if you want an organized and clutter-free vibe in your workspace, then fluorite is a great crystal to have on your desk. A white quartz crystal is great for all kinds of spaces and areas. It helps in uplifting, positive vibrations and cleansing the environment.

Tiger's eye or aventurine attracts wealth and prosperity. So, place one or both in your living room or business space. Orange crystals like carnelian, citrine, sodalite, and others imbue intimacy in the surroundings and are excellent for placing in bedrooms.

In addition to healing and cleansing benefits, crystals are great for adding some oomph and oeuvre to your décor. Their beauty and shine can enhance the aesthetics of any room.

4. ***Place a suitable crystal over your goal and dream lists***

First, create a dream list in the present tense and not in the future tense. For example, don't write, "I want to be healthy and strong." Write, "I am healthy, strong, and full of vitality." Suppose this is your top desire because you have been plagued by various physical illnesses in the recent past.

Take a crystal whose vibrational energy is in sync with your goal. For example, green aventurine or onyx are excellent for building energy and vitality. So, fold the paper on which you have written down your intentions for strength and vitality, and place the chosen crystal over it. You can place it on the altar (if you have one). If you don't have an altar, you can place it anywhere where it will not be disturbed.

The crystal behaves like a battery and charges up your intention, and direct the universal energy to manifest your outcomes.

5. ***Use crystals to cleanse and clear up your personal energy and/or aura***

If your physical space is dusty and unclean, don't you use a brush to clear up the area, and make it clean again? Some crystals work just like brushes or brooms to cleanse and clear up negativities trapped in the field of your personal aura.

For example, a selenite wand can identify, and pull out negative energy patterns from the energy field of your personal aura to neutralize and dissolve them into nothingness. Wave the selenite wand all over your body in a brushing action. Keep the wand about a foot away from your body while doing this cleansing action.

Another effective way of cleansing your personal aura is to direct all frenetic and harsh energies to black crystals such as obsidian, smoky quartz, or tourmaline. Hold one such crystal in your hand, and consciously transfer all the negativities to the crystal. When you have done this, place the crystal in bright sunlight to allow the trapped negativities to evaporate into the atmosphere.

6. ***Put crystal essences into your drinking water***

Crystal essences or gem elixirs are a convenient way to harness the benefits of the vibrational energies of crystals. They can be made easily and stored for later use. Moreover, these crystal essences are also found in stores.

You can use one, two, or more crystals to make your gem elixir. A combination of crystals results in an advantageous blend of all the synergies of the gemstones used. The total synergy of vibrations of many crystals is invariably more than the sum of all of them. The following steps help you to prepare the gem elixir at home:

Required items - Get the following items ready before you start the preparation process.

- Choose the crystal(s) you want to make the elixir of. You can include similar types of crystals (for examples, different types of quartzes) to enhance the charge of the essence.
- Two containers made of glass or any other food-safe materials; the sizes should be such that one should fit into the other with a little gap available between the two. For

example, you can take a glass jar that fits into a glass bowl with some room available between the two.

- Two dark-colored bottles of different sizes
- A glass stopper
- Distilled water or spring water
- Any variety of vinegar or vodka (80 proof or higher) – this is the preservative
- A calm and steady mind with a clear intention to create a powerful gem elixir

How to make crystal essence - You can make this potion outdoors or indoors as long as you get sufficient sunlight or moonlight for the process. You can also use your personal space or altar (if you have one) to prepare the elixir.

- First, clear, cleanse, and charge the crystals.
- Next, center yourself, and create the right intention with prayers and breathing techniques.
- Say your intention aloud so that the divine energies and the crystals prepare themselves to help you in your endeavor.
- Place the large container in the determined space.
- Place the small container inside the large container. Ensure the position is stable, and that it will not topple over.

- Fill as much of water as you can into the larger container ensuring that nothing falls into the small container.
- Arrange the crystals in the small container.
- State your intent again, and the crystals and water in the designated place for at least four hours.
- Then, gently pour out the crystal-charged water from the large container into the larger of the two bottles. Pour the water until it is halfway full.
- Pour vodka or vinegar until the bottle is full. This preservative helps to 'fix' the vibrational energy of the crystals in the water.
- Transfer a small amount of this elixir into the smaller of the two bottles for immediate use. You can use distilled water or spring water to dilute this elixir if you want.
- Thank the crystal(s) and the divine energies for helping you create the gem elixir.

Store the larger bottle of this amazing gem elixir safely for future use. You can refrigerate the crystal essence for a few days. But, you must use it quickly. Alternately, you can make crystal essence in the same way in smaller quantities for immediate use in which case you do not need to add any preservatives. It is important not to put crystals directly into the water as the soft ones will dissolve.

If you don't want to go through the rigmarole of making your own elixir, you can use store-bought ones too. Add a few drops into your drinking water and you are, in effect, bringing the crystals' vibration into your own vibrational energy, which can result in powerful changes for you.

7. *Create crystal grids*

If you have multiple crystals, then you can make a crystal grid to create positive changes in your life. Making the effort to create the grid itself can result in positive changes. However, you can get added benefits if you let loose your creativity, and make a crystal that resonates with the vibrational powers of all the crystals involved in the grid. Additionally, the Universal Divine energy will also open doors for you.

You can use a geometric pattern of your choice, though the 'mandala' is one of the most powerful and popular grid pattern used by experts in the crystal world. The geometric pattern also adds its own to the potent mix of crystal energies. In fact, if made correctly and creatively, the energy of a crystal grid is almost palpable.

How to create a crystal grid – Use the following steps to create your own crystal grid in your home:

- A suitable undisturbed space in your home.
- A small piece of paper in which you have written your intent.
- A central crystal; typically, this central piece would be a crystal point that would help in transmitting your intention out into the universe. However, any good crystal will also work.
- Tumbled stone crystals whose vibrational energies are aligned with your purpose.
- A crystal grid garment or cloth; this is optional though it enhances the power of the grid.

First, determine your intention for the crystal grid. What do you want?

- Do you want to attract prosperity, wealth, and abundance?
- Do you want health and fitness?
- Do you want peace of mind?
- Do you want improved creativity?

- Do you want to attract love?

The more specific your intentions are, the easier it is to choose the right crystals for the grid. You can create a crystal grid for any intention of your choice. There are no restrictions at all.

- Next, choose the crystals that are aligned with your intentions. For example, for prosperity and abundance, you will need gold and green crystals such as citrine, aventurine, pyrite, etc. For health, you will need purple and blue gemstones like Angelite, sodalite, fluorite, etc. There are no right or wrong answers for the type of crystals you use for your crystal grid. Choose the gemstones that you feel drawn to, and feel intuitively positive.
- Cleanse and recharge your crystals. Cleanse the crystal grid space too.
- Spread your crystal grid cloth, and in its center, place a piece of paper with your intentions written down.
- Next, state your intention aloud.
- Start placing the crystals in the grid beginning from the outward boundary moving towards the center. As you put each crystal in its place, ensure you are visualizing or thinking about your intentions.

- Lastly, place the central crystal on top of the written intention.
- Now, activate the crystal grid. For this, take a crystal point, and draw an invisible line running through all the crystals on the grid. Think of the 'connecting the dots' game you used to play as a child.

With this, your crystal grid is activated, and its energy will begin to do its magic in your life. For maximum benefit, please keep your crystal grid intact for a minimum of 40 days.

8. *Use the power of a crystal to heal or open a chakra*

If you know that one or more of your chakras needs healing or there is a blockage of energy there, you can use crystals for this purpose too. You must choose a crystal corresponding to the color associated with the particular chakra. Here is a quick guide for each of the seven chakras:

The root chakra (the first chakra) is associated with the color red, and the crystals that work best are red garnet, smoky quartz, red jasper, hematite, etc.

The sacral chakra (the second chakra) is connected with the color orange, and crystal for this include carnelian, amber, orange calcite, goldstone, tiger's eye, etc.

The solar plexus chakra (the third chakra) is linked to the color yellow. The crystals for healing or unblocking the energy in the third chakra include yellow jade, pyrite, rutilated quartz, etc.

The heart chakra (the fourth chakra) is connected to two colors, pink and green. The heart chakra crystals include amazonite, emerald, green calcite, aventurine, rose quartz, etc.

The throat chakra (the fifth chakra) is linked to the color blue. The crystals for the throat chakra include kyanite, Angelite, apatite, sodalite, aquamarine, etc.

The third eye chakra (the sixth one) is associated with the purple color. Crystals that help in the healing of the sixth chakra include fluorite, amethyst, charoite, iolite, and more.

The last of the seven chakras is the crown chakra which is connected with the color violet and white. Crystals that work well this chakra are clear quartz, blue lace agate, ametrine, lepidolite, and more.

9. ***Bury crystals under the earth to create a protective and/or empowering boundary***

You can bury quartz crystals at the four corners of a plot of land or any other space for protection as well as empowerment. For the protection of plots of land, it is best to choose large-sized crystals. The bigger the size of the crystals, the better protection your space gets.

It is important to clear, cleanse, and recharge the crystals before burying them. Also, transfer the power of your intention to the crystals. When you bury them, remember to keep the pointed side facing upwards for effective dissipation of negative energies and also to direct the attention of the universal energy for protection.

10. ***Place crystals all over your body***

Placing crystals directly on your body has a completely different effect from that of holding them in your hands. For example, if you are looking to unblock the energies in a particular chakra, then take the chakra corresponding to that chakra, and place it directly on the body part connected to that chakra. This approach stirs up the energy vibrations in and around the chakra region and works with your emotions for healing and creating positivity.

For example, place an aventurine on your heart chakra to give and receive love. Place a quartz crystal on your crown chakra to receive guidance and enlightenment from the divine. If you meditate by placing an amethyst stone on your third eye chakra, your ability to enter a deeper level of consciousness increases.

Work with all the different ways mentioned in this chapter. Each situation calls for a different healing method. Additionally, you must include your intuition to check out what works best for you and your needs. Try all of them, and you will realize that some of the methods work brilliantly while some others give you average results. Experiment a lot, and don't forget to learn from each experiment.

Conclusion

The power of crystals lies in their vibrational energies in their molecular system that has been set up within their system over millions of year. The color, the shape, and the property of each crystal and gemstone have been formed over millennia. They hold the natural energies of the Earth and the universe. The deeper crystals were buried in the depths of the Earth (thanks to natural pressure and heat applied on them), and more energy was accumulated in their molecular system.

The structure of the crystal system is such that the vibrational energy trapped within it can be aligned to optimize healing and well-being for the holder of the crystal. Crystals and gemstones work with various frequencies of vibrational energies and can use the resulting energy resonance to help you achieve your dreams and desires.

Depending on your thoughts, needs and willpower, the frequency of the vibrational energy of the crystal combines and interacts with the energy of your personal aura to help you realize your goals and intentions.

Every crystal's power is unique. The uniqueness is not restricted to one type of crystal, but every stone is different from another one. There will be similarities in the way they function. For example, two pieces of clear quartz can help bring clarity for you. However, each piece will work in its own unique way to perform this function.

The uniqueness of each crystal is so well defined that if you lose or damage a gemstone, then finding another one that gives out the exact same outcome as the lost one is impossible. You will simply have to accept something that works similarly.

A final point to remember is that crystals and gemstones cannot work their magic on their own. They need the energy of your powerful intention to help you achieve your dreams. Without your inner power, personal aura, and mental strength, crystals and gemstones will remain decorative items. So, delve deep, find your power, and multiply and magnify it with the help of crystals and gemstones.

Resources

http://www.crystalage.com/crystal_information/crystal_history/

https://www.mindbodygreen.com/0-16394/how-to-choose-a-healing-crystal-thats-right-for-you.html

https://www.mindbodygreen.com/0-91/The-7-Chakras-for-Beginners.html

https://www.mindbodygreen.com/articles/how-to-recognize-when-the-universe-is-giving-you-a-sign

http://www.chakras.info/chakra-colors/

https://www.ethanlazzerini.com/crystals-beginners/

https://www.mindbodygreen.com/0-14044/10-crystals-that-will-make-you-healthier-happier.html

https://www.energymuse.com

https://www.gaia.com/article/crystal-care-clearing-cleansing-charging-your-crystals

http://www.thatcrystalsite.com/take-care-crystals-stones/

https://meanings.crystalsandjewelry.com/how-to-make-gem-elixirs-or-crystal-essences/

https://tesswhitehurst.com/the-10-best-ways-to-use-crystals-in-your-magical-and-spiritual-work/

https://www.energymuse.com/blog/using-healing-crystals/

www.ingramcontent.com/pod-product-compliance
Lightning Source LLC
LaVergne TN
LVHW041744190726
843493LV00008B/2444